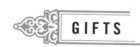

30 DAYS OF HOPE

FOR STRENGTH IN CHRONIC ILLNESS

ELIZABETH EVANS

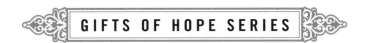

GIFTS OF HOPE SERIES

30 DAYS OF HOPE
FOR STRENGTH IN CHRONIC ILLNESS

ELIZABETH EVANS

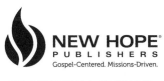

NEW HOPE®
PUBLISHERS
Gospel-Centered. Missions-Driven.

BIRMINGHAM, ALABAMA

New Hope® Publishers
PO Box 12065
Birmingham, AL 35202-2065
NewHopePublishers.com
New Hope Publishers is a division of WMU®.

Library of Congress Cataloging-in-Publication Data:
Names: Evans, G. Elizabeth, 1966-
Title: 30 days of hope for strength in chronic illness / G. Elizabeth Evans.
Other titles: Thirty days of hope for strength in chronic illness
Description: Birmingham, AL : New Hope Publishers, 2016.
Identifiers: LCCN 2015039903 | ISBN 9781596694651 (sc)
Subjects: LCSH: Chronically ill–Religious life. | Chronic
    diseases–Religious aspects–Christianity. | Cystic
    fibrosis–Patients–Religious life.
Classification: LCC BV4910 .E93 2016 | DDC 248.8/61–dc23 LC record
available at http://lccn.loc.gov/2015039903

All scripture quotations, unless otherwise indicated, are taken from the Holy Bible, New International Version®, NIV®. Copyright © 1973, 1978, 1984, 2011 by Biblica, Inc.™ Used by permission of Zondervan. All rights reserved worldwide. www.zondervan.com The "NIV" and "New International Version" are trademarks registered in the United States Patent and Trademark Office by Biblica, Inc.™

Scripture quotations marked (NKJV) are taken from the New King James Version®. Copyright © 1982 by Thomas Nelson. Used by permission. All rights reserved.

Scripture quotations marked (NLT) are taken from the Holy Bible, New Living Translation, copyright © 1996, 2004, 2007, 2013 by Tyndale House Foundation. Used by permission of Tyndale House Publishers, Inc., Carol Stream, Illinois 60188. All rights reserved.

Lyrics from "Grace Greater than Our Sin" (1910) by Julia Harriet Johnston on page 41.

ISBN-10: 1-59669-465-3
ISBN-13: 978-1-59669-465-1

N164105 • 0216 • 1M1

I DEDICATE THIS WORK IN MEMORY OF

KYMBERLY JOYCE TASCOTT,

MY MOST BELOVED FRIEND AND SISTER IN CHRIST.

Kym and I were best friends and roomies in our early twenties. She, as well as I, was diagnosed with cystic fibrosis in early childhood. At the age of 23, Kym lost her life to CF. From her, I learned so much about living, laughing, and loving amid the daily struggles that are encountered when living with chronic and eventual terminal illness. My life is forever changed and my heart will forever ache this side of heaven. Until we meet again, Kym, this is for you.

TABLE OF CONTENTS

I WANT TO THANK MY HUSBAND, DAVID, for being my greatest fan and cheerleader. When I have gotten off course and felt as though writing may not be my calling, he always encourages me. He has stood by me in this journey of life and chronic illness. He always is refreshed and ready to cheer me on, whether in my battle with cystic fibrosis (CF), my writing, or my relationship with the Lord. I am truly blessed. *Thank you, David. I love you.*

I ALSO WANT TO HONOR MY MOTHER and her fight for and with me in life. Her unwillingness to hear what the doctors told her about life expectancy, quality of life, and what the eventual outcome would be. For all the tears she shed over me, for me, and with me. For her unceasing prayers. For the strength she has always shown in the midst of constant illness and complications in the lives of her children due to CF. For her trust in and dependence on God for our every need and how she taught me, by example, in Him alone is my hope. For her love that has always been constant and unconditional. *Thank you, Mommy, I love you so much.*

"Her children arise and call her blessed."

—Proverbs 31:28

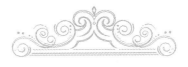

PREFACE

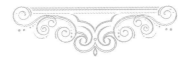

A T THE age of 18 months, I was diagnosed with cystic fibrosis. CF, as it is referred to, is a genetic disease affecting about 30,000 children and adults in the United States and 15,000 in the United Kingdom. CF causes an over-production of thick and sticky mucus throughout the entire body. The lungs are the most affected, but other parts of the body the disease attacks include the endocrine system, the digestive system, the sweat glands, the sinuses, and the liver.

A normal day, when I am well enough to be at home rather than in the hospital, consists of three 45-minute chest physical therapies, 11 to 12 aerosol medications, and anywhere from 25 to 30 oral medications.

The chest physical therapy is done in two ways. In one I am connected to a machine that literally shakes me to try to dislodge the thick, sticky mucus from my lungs.

Sometimes my husband becomes the therapy machine, pounding on my back, sides and chest for the same purpose. The aerosol medications are taken throughout the day, usually with five in the morning, one or two in the afternoon, and five in the evening. These medications include a bronchodilator, a long-acting steroid, a medication made just for CF patients that thins the mucus, and an inhaled antibiotic. The oral medications have various purposes, helping my body do what it doesn't seem to want to do on its own: control asthma and reflux, help digest foods, and fight infection.

When I become ill enough to be hospitalized, I receive more physical therapies, additional aerosols, plus high-powered IV antibiotics. These hospitalizations last a minimum of 14 days and usually, for me, 21 to 30 days. As I have become older, my hospitalizations have increased in both frequency and length.

At the time I was diagnosed, average life expectancy for CF patients was only ten years. However, my parents were told that I would not live to be three. By the grace of God, I am now 48. Even though I've had a very blessed and full life, I am now facing a double lung transplant to prolong my life. The road has not always been easy, but I love adventure. Growing up, I faced dying at a young age. This caused me to learn very young that life was not to be taken for granted. Life is meant to be savored and lived to the fullest—no matter your circumstances.

My passion and desire is to encourage everyone to live life to the fullest, no matter their health or prognosis. Each day that I am granted is for a purpose. I want to honor the Lord with my life and all that He allows me to do for Him.

As you read this book, I pray that you will be blessed, that the Holy Spirit will speak to you in your particular circumstances, that you will recognize His wooing of your spirit, and that you will be drawn closer to the Lord.

In Christ,

Beth

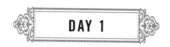

DAY 1

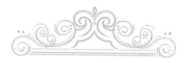

GRACE FOR THE JOURNEY

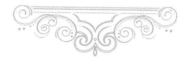

*So let us come boldly to the throne
of our gracious God.
There we will receive his mercy,
and we will find grace to help us
when we need it most.*

—HEBREWS 4:16 NLT

GRACE. God's unmerited favor. We cannot earn it, nor can we lose the unmerited favor of God. What an awesome gift! The gift of grace for this journey through life. No matter where you are in your struggles with whatever illness you face physically, mentally, or emotionally, the grace of God covers you. Sometimes that grace is an invisible veil, but at other times the covering of grace has seemed almost tangible to me.

Aside from living with chronic illness, I have had experiences I could not have made it through emotionally without grace from God. Just in the past 13 years, there have been especially trying times of heartache and disillusionment. I have experienced the deaths of both my husband's parents. I lost my own father in 2007 from cancer. Only 25 days after his diagnosis, the family gathered at his funeral. Besides my own grief, it was hard to watch my mom agonize over the death of her sweetheart of 48 years.

While it is natural to lose family members from the generation above us, in 2010 we lost our ten-month-old grandchild who had been born with three major heart defects. As parents we have also experienced the devastating decisions made by some of our adult children, decisions contrary to the Word of God and the training they received. And we have had the same anxiety of all parents when one son, who is a sergeant in the Army, was deployed to Afghanistan and Iraq multiple times.

These difficulties are just part of my everyday life. If we could sit and talk, your list might be longer than mine. That is why I am so thankful that each of us can come boldly before God's throne of grace. As today's Scripture says, He promises to bestow grace upon us to help us with everything we need.

Although this book is about dealing with chronic illness, all our needs are not physical. We may need grace to deliver us from depression—to help get us out of bed in the morning to face the day ahead of us. We may need His grace to calm our emotions and our nerves when we are racked with fear and worry. What an encouraging promise we find in 1 Peter 5:12 (NLT): "My purpose in writing is to encourage you and assure you that what you are experiencing is truly part of God's grace for you. Stand firm in this grace."

At times this grace may seem almost tangible to you, too. You could receive a direct word to your spirit through a comforting Scripture verse. Or God may send someone to minister directly to you. He might open a door of opportunity you thought was closed. Be encouraged and remember that even when grace does not come in the way you expect, it is still there. His peace that passes all understanding (Philippians 4:7) is a gift of His grace for the journey. His love that is all-encompassing is a gift of His grace for the journey. His compassions that never fail and His faithfulness are gifts of grace for the journey.

Whatever your need is today, go boldly before His throne of grace with your requests, and you will have everything you need to get you through this day.

DEAR LORD,

Thank You that You have already provided what I need to get through this day. Thank You for grace for my journey. Lord, I pray that even when that gift of grace may not be what I am expecting, I will be mindful of Your grace. I praise You for Your gift of grace in my life. Amen.

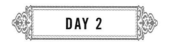

DAY 2

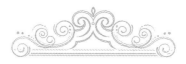

JUST ENOUGH LIGHT

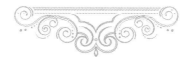

For we walk by faith, not by sight.

—2 CORINTHIANS 5:7 NKJV

STORMIE Omartian wrote a popular book called, *Just Enough Light for the Step I'm On.* I read it at a time when I needed its message, and it ministered to me greatly. Little did I know then how many times I would return to that book, realizing each time how well it describes how God graciously lights only the step we are on.

When the children of Israel left Egypt and were led into the wilderness, they were told they were headed to the Promised Land. However, if they had known it was going to take 40 years and that some generations would not enter the Promised Land, but instead would die in the wilderness due to their unbelief, they might not have left Egypt. They knew where they had been—in bondage. And they knew where they were headed—to the Promised Land—but the details were left to God.

When I think of this with regard to my health, I know that it is by God's grace alone that I can see where I am physically, but not where I am headed. After many serious complications related to my cystic fibrosis, I can look back and realize why He did not show me the future. Oh, how thankful I have been over and over! How thankful my mom and dad were and my husband is now that they cannot foresee what's coming. Instead of living in dread of what might be coming, we can live in the here and now and know that God's grace will see us through. It's because of His loving grace that He only lights the step we are on currently. Wow . . . how amazing is that? Trust me, I usually like to know where I am headed, but with my health I have learned that it's much better that I have no idea. As my granddaughter would say, "It would freak me out!" No light? No problem. I have no reason to freak out because of God's grace.

Light for just the step you are on also keeps you from constantly looking back, which could cause you to stumble. When we stay in the light and focus on that alone, we cannot be held captive by fear or emotions related to the journey we have already traveled. How so like God! Focus on where He has you today—where your health is today. Not what it might have been or where it could end up. God gives grace for today, to live today to the fullest and to deal with whatever issues your health brings you.

Whatever step you are on physically, when you find yourself wanting to anticipate the next step, don't. Only as you step onto it will it become illuminated. The light remains until you move to the next step. Your health may change, maybe often and vastly; however, God's grace never does!

DEAR LORD,

Thank You for only lighting the step I am on. What grace You show me day-to-day, month-to-month, and year-to-year as my health changes. Your grace does not waver. Lord, may I find contentment in the light of Your grace. Amen.

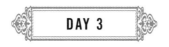

DAY 3

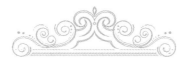

NEW MERCIES
EACH MORNING

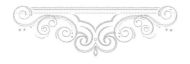

*The faithful love of the L*ord *never ends!*
His mercies never cease. Great is his faithfulness;
his mercies begin afresh each morning.

—Lamentations 3:22–23 NLT

EVER notice how problems seem much bigger at night than they do in the morning? Many times as problems arise during the day, and as my husband and I begin to discuss them, they seem to grow. Whether they are dealing with our family, our finances, or our health, no matter how bleak things seemed when we went to bed, they seem so much smaller and better in the morning. I find that is true even when I am feeling discouraged about what is going on in my body, no matter how sick I may be at the time. Each morning brings new mercies. New perspective. New encouragement.

When the children of Israel were in the wilderness, God rained down manna fresh every morning. They could not store up the manna because it would rot. They had to trust Him to provide for them a fresh supply each day. We cannot store up His provision in our life. We must trust Him on a daily basis also, realizing that whatever needs we have or are ever going to have are provided.

Living with CF all my life, I have lost many friends to CF. Because of those losses, I've always known that I might die from complications of CF. Over the last ten years, double lung transplant has been found to be a life-lengthening procedure for those living with CF. I have had several friends in the past few years who have undergone transplant. I never thought I would consider that option. As I have shared with many who ask, I know this side of the coin (living with the disease) but I am not too sure about the other side.

Due to the decline in my lung function this year, which is a natural progression of the disease, I was referred to the transplant team at my local hospital for evaluation. I found out very quickly I had been turned down. Just as problems often do, the answer of "no" began to echo ominously over me. I prayed for direction as I trusted in God and His will for my life. As I soon discovered, He had already made provision for me at another hospital in another state. Within only a few weeks from the time I was denied a transplant by one hospital, I was accepted into the pretransplant program at another. My need had been provided for before I knew I needed it. I only needed to trust in that provision.

I cannot say that everything you think you need will be provided or that you will like being in need. (Most of us don't.) You may be hurting. You may be broken in spirit. You may feel as though your world is crashing down around you. You may feel hopeless regarding your physical needs or your emotional needs. Whatever you need and however you are feeling, remember that God's mercies are new every morning. Just as the manna rained down, so do His provisions for you. Today is a new day. Tomorrow is a new day. New mercies every morning!

Dear Lord,

Thank You for Your mercies being new every day. Thank You for Your provision for my needs. I praise You for going before me and making provisions even when I am not yet aware of my needs. Lord, may I always trust in Your provisions in my life. Amen.

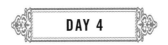

DAY 4

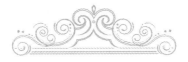

GRACE
FOR TODAY

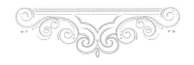

But whatever I am now,
it is all because God poured out
his special favor on me—
and not without results.
For I have worked harder
than any of the other apostles;
yet it was not I but God
who was working through me by his grace.

—1 Corinthians 15:10 NLT

A PRIL 15, 2013, began as any other Monday. I had errands to run: grocery shopping, pick up something at the drug store, and a few extra stops. I was more tired than usual, the weather and pollen made it more difficult to breathe, but I was doing OK. I just had to push a little harder, but that often made up my "normal" day.

However, as it so happened, that day was anything but normal. It will forever be remembered as the Monday that the Boston Marathon was bombed. In one instant, lives were changed forever! Just as on 9/11, those affected had done nothing to place themselves in vulnerable positions. They were just going about their normal duties of everyday life.

Normal life, for those of us struggling with chronic illness, is made up of doctor's appointments, tests, test results, and treatments. We seem to grow accustomed to change. Our normal is looked upon as abnormal by most people. Our lives can change in an instant. One call from the doctor, one bad day after another, test results you'd rather not get. Yet, no matter how bad our day may be, we are never outside the bounds of God's grace. He gives grace for every day. Grace for whatever life may throw at us. Grace for the good news and the bad.

The grace that enveloped me as I ran my errands, feeling yucky and breathing heavily is the same grace available to the families directly and indirectly affected by the tragedy in Boston. The same grace that carries us all through every day. God's grace knows no limits or boundaries! It is the same for everyone in every situation. It is more than sufficient to carry us through whatever we encounter. God's grace! What peace is spoken to my spirit, no matter what is happening in my body, in my family, or in the world around me. God's grace is more than enough.

Whatever we face on a daily basis, large or small, bringing abounding joy or absolute devastation, God's grace is with us. Remind yourself often of His sustaining grace. Praise God for His grace. Pray to become keenly aware of His grace in every moment of every day, in every situation and circumstance. Learn to live in His grace daily!

DEAR LORD,

No matter what I may face today, may I recognize Your grace for every situation. May I stay close to You, in a place of praise and thankfulness for Your sustaining grace. I thank You now for Your grace and peace. Amen.

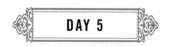

DAY 5

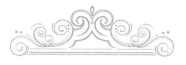

GOD'S GOT THIS

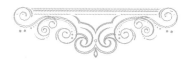

Sing for joy, O heavens! Rejoice, O earth!
Burst into song, O mountains!
For the LORD has comforted his people and will have
compassion on them in their suffering.

—ISAIAH 49:13 NLT

MY HUSBAND, David, my mom, and I were traveling through the Smoky Mountains of Tennessee on our way to Durham, North Carolina. As we crossed into North Carolina, the beauty of the mountain range was amazing.

I began to think about how the awe in which we observe the creation of our God is totally opposite to the awe, and even fear, that we experience when we face mountainous circumstances in our lives. God uses mountainous circumstances to mature us and to help build our trust in Him. He also uses us to minister to others during and after we have faced similar situations in our lives. I know that with one word He could cause those mountains of circumstance to move and be cast into the sea, and He has at times. But more often I find that the mountains stay put, and I grow in the midst of the journey to overcome struggles.

Driving along the highway with praise music playing, we were all singing. I remember looking at the mountains surrounding us, but I was seeing them through the eyes of my spirit. I began thanking God for them. Thanking Him for the beauty they bring to the landscape. Just as He uses the struggles in our lives, to bring beauty out of ashes (Isaiah 61:3).

My thoughts turned to the reason we were traveling to North Carolina. We were on our way to Duke Medical Clinic for me to be evaluated for a double lung transplant.

I was not worried but quite overwhelmed by all that could be ahead of me and our family. Then I noticed the road went directly through the mountains. We were surrounded by the mountains on both sides. Huge walls of rock and slate seemed to close in on us as we drove along. They had cut the roadway directly through the mountain. Not over, not around, but straight *through*. At that moment, I felt the Lord whisper to my spirit, "I've got this! Do not worry about what lies ahead or how I get you there, just know that I will make a way." He knew the mountain of circumstance that I would see ahead, but He already had cleared the way.

In my travels to other parts of the United States and the world, I have noticed that every mountain range is vastly different. The way they arc or roll, the heights they climb to, the amount of landscape they consume. The colors, shapes, and even the terrain are all different. That is also true of the circumstances we face in our lives. Just as the needs of mountain climbers vary from climb to climb, so do our needs. The route may change, the time it takes to reach the top may vary, and the level of endurance needed may increase. However, in each of our journeys, we can trust the Lord as our guide. He will supply all our needs, and give us more than enough grace (strength, patience, endurance . . .) for whatever we may face along the journey.

He's got this!

DEAR LORD,

You know that I look at my circumstances through natural eyes. Help me to see my situation through spiritual eyes. Lord, guide me, as I trust in Your leading. I know that You have supplied all my needs and You have already made a way! Lord, I take comfort and find peace in knowing that You have got this. Amen.

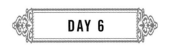

DAY 6

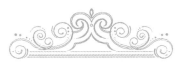

GIFTS
OF GRACE

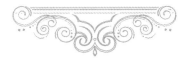

*And my God will meet all your needs
according to the riches of his glory in Christ Jesus.*

—Philippians 4:19

Due to being in the hospital so much, I have had many visitors, especially from my church family. Through these visits God has blessed me with a very special gift of grace by forming a relationship between an elderly gentleman and me. My gift arrives every Monday and is wrapped up in a tall, 80-year-old man—an associate pastor at our church—with a smile that radiates warmth and joy as he begins to talk about his Lord and Savior Jesus Christ. He reminds me so much of my grandfather with his simple yet profoundly genuine love of others and his humble spirit as he approaches me but, even more so, as he approaches the Lord in prayer.

We found common ground very quickly when we both shared that we love life, enjoying it to the fullest, and that we absolutely don't like being slowed down—much less stopped. The time flies as the conversation flows and all too soon he has to go. I feel a sense of bittersweetness. While I hate to see him go, I know the best part is yet to come. He drops to his knees and begins to pray. That is when I feel the Spirit of the Lord fill the room.

One day another minister from church came by to check on me. As he entered my room, he gave me a beautiful butterfly that lights up. He told me that my special friend had sent it to me. I wanted to cry. It was like a hug from God. Just like the hug from God that I felt every Monday, my special gift of grace. I keep that butterfly on my desk and reach for it when I need to feel that hug.

God is so awesome! May we always be thankful for the amazing grace gifts He places in our lives at just the right time and in just the right way. May we never misappropriate such gifts when they are given. May we never cease to be amazed by the love of our Heavenly Father and the depths He will go to as He seeks to demonstrate His love for us.

HEAVENLY FATHER,

I pray that the eyes and ears of my spirit will recognize Your gifts of grace. I pray that as I go about my daily life and all the struggles I may encounter, that I will always yield myself unto You, a willing vessel. And may I also become a gift of grace in someone else's life! Amen.

Gifts of Grace

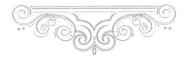

God's gifts of grace wash over me,
From the words I hear to the faces I see;
Encouraging words so loving and dear,
Faces filled with sunshine, joy, and cheer.

Hearts that are open, accepting, and true,
Hearts full of love ordained only of You.

The tears of a friend or the laughter of a child,
The warmth of a touch, a hug, or a smile.

Compassion I see in the eyes of the one I love,
So understanding and enduring
it could only be from above.

I am astonished when I take note of all that I see,
Knowing when You gave these gifts
You were thinking of me.

"Grace, grace, God's grace,
Grace that is greater than all my sin.
Grace, grace, God's grace
Grace that will pardon and cleanse within."
—Grace Greater Than Our Sin

My PRAYER *is that others, through a touch or a word or a simple smiling face, would truly comprehend Your love as they recognize Your awesome gifts of grace.*

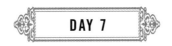

DAY 7

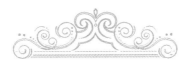

RUN TO HIM

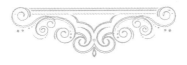

The LORD is my light and my salvation;
Whom shall I fear?
The LORD is the strength of my life;
Of whom shall I be afraid?

—PSALM 27:1 NKJV

ECAUSE I have lived my entire life dealing with cystic fibrosis and all it encompasses, many have told me that I am strong. They see the piles of medications I take daily, the hours of chest physical therapy and aerosol medication treatments to clear the mucus out of my lungs, and the numerous hospitalizations every year. They see my health declining as I get older. They also see that among all the physical struggles, I love my life and I live every day to the fullest. They do not see the broken little girl who runs home to Daddy God when I am hurting. He picks me up, dusts me off, and puts me back on my way, but I go running back to Him again and again and again. He is my strength. My comforter. My peace. I do cry. I do hurt. I get disappointed. I get discouraged. However, I have a haven to run to. I have a loving Heavenly Father who will scoop me up, and let me rest in His lap of love while He dries my every tear and refills me with His strength.

One of my all-time favorite songs is "The Warrior" by Twyla Paris. The chorus of the song paints such a vivid picture of my relationship with God. The song is a conversation between her and God as she relates to Him how others see her versus how she really is. The lyrics tell the story of how, throughout all her struggles, others view her as a warrior: strong, mighty, and fearless. But they only see the strength that comes from God. They do not see how she struggles within as she faces each trial. She tells God that what others don't see is that the warrior runs home, drops her sword, and cries in the lap of the Lord—that inside, the warrior is really a child. That's my life. Is that your life?

Whatever you may face. When your strength fails and you fall to your knees. When you feel as though you cannot carry on. When fear tries to fill your mind. When the daily struggles of chronic illness seem to overwhelm you. When others see your strength but you feel as though you are falling apart—*run to Him!* Go running home! Let Him pick you up and hold you in His love and grace. Allow Him to comfort you and restore your strength and peace.

Run, run, run to Him!

DEAR LORD,

I run to You! This little girl needs You to pick me up, hold me close, and dry my tears. Others may see my strength, but I know my weakness. I feel so weak and overwhelmed. I need Your peace and Your strength. I am running to You, Lord! Amen.

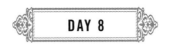

DAY 8

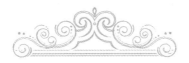

FIGHT THE GOOD FIGHT

Joshua said to them,
"Do not be afraid; do not be discouraged.
Be strong and courageous.
*This is what the L*ORD *will do to all*
the enemies you are going to fight."

—JOSHUA 10:25

NUMEROUS times a year I am hospitalized just to keep my health at a level that I have good quality of life. In the last three years it seems like I have been in the hospital more than at home. Not long ago, I found myself returning to the hospital after being home for only one week. I got a weird virus that caused my asthma to kick in like gangbusters. I tried to fight it out at home, but after seven days when I was still no better, the return to the hospital, or as I call it, Club Med, was inevitable.

I would love to say that I am so strong that this was not devastating, but it was. I was feeling so good when I left the hospital that for something as minor as a cold or virus to have knocked me down so fast and furiously was quite discouraging. Yet, I refused to give in to CF, sickness, discouragement, or depression. I was, and still am, determined to fight the good fight! I see so many sad situations being in and around the hospital as much as I am. So many people do not and cannot enjoy the quality of life that I do. I am constantly reminded how truly blessed I am.

Even with all the challenges, I would not change a thing nor would I ever trade for someone else's problems. God calls us to be content where we are, in whatever state we may find ourselves in. Not looking at what once was, nor focusing on what might or could have been. Be content in your journey, your race, your fight.

Each of us has our own struggles and issues in life. Sickness, disease, depression, anxiety. Whatever your battle is, take heart, do not be discouraged nor dismayed. Fight the good fight! In the midst of your worst day or trying situation, look around and you will see how blessed you really are. Smell the roses. Live. Laugh. Love. Each day is a new and blessed gift from God our Father. Continue to fight the good fight, and give God the glory as you gain each victory!

DEAR LORD,

You alone know what real battles I face on a daily basis. I pray that as I encounter each new battle, I will look to You for my strength and courage. Please forgive me when I do not give You praise in every victory, whether great or small. May I bring honor to You as I am encouraged to fight the good fight. Amen.

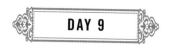

DAY 9

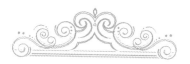

EMOTIONAL AMBUSH

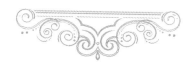

You keep track of all my sorrows.
You have collected all my tears in your bottle.
You have recorded each one in your book.

—Psalm 56:8 NLT

Y AUNT was the one who introduced me to the term *emotional ambush*. Emotional ambush refers to a time when you are doing well, living life as a participant rather than an onlooker, feeling good and then . . . boom, out of the blue . . . a situation causes hurt or brings up painful memories. The ambush may be related to your physical condition or psychological feelings of inadequacy. Any day, any time, and without reason, you can fall prey to this kind of ambush.

The first time this happened to me was at a family gathering for a celebration. Just before everyone left, we began making traditional group pictures. The siblings gathered around their mom, my grandmother, who was 94. The grandchildren, then the great-grands, and then the great-great-grands. The last picture to be taken was of the spouses of my grandmother's children, because they were considered children also. I was one of the ones taking pictures and, as the "out-laws" gathered around Grandmommy, I held up my camera ready to snap the photo. Then *bam*, out of nowhere, I realized that my daddy was missing from the photo. I had to leave the room! My daddy has been gone for five years, yet I was ambushed by the emotion of how much I miss him.

No matter what causes your emotional ambush, catching you off guard and bringing you to your knees, you only have to look up for your restoration. God is never caught off guard. He keeps track of all your sorrows. He knows your needs before you ask. He knows your innermost fears, questions, confusion, and pain. Only He can restore you emotionally, physically, and mentally. Surrender your emotions and fears to Him.

Whatever your emotional turmoil may be today, remember that your Heavenly Father is your comfort. Allow His peace to drive away your fear. There's not one tear you can shed without His notice. How precious to know that He collects all our tears in a bottle. He knows every tear we shed and why. He keeps track of them. What a loving Father!

DEAR LORD,

You know my heart for You created me. You know and understand my hurts as well as my joys. I praise You, Father, that You love me with a love I cannot even fathom. You know my thoughts, the number of hairs on my head, and You collect all my tears in Your bottle. Thank You for lovingly embracing me when I feel ambushed emotionally. You are my strength. Amen.

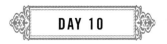

DAY 10

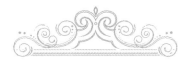

BITTER
OR BETTER?

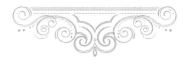

When they came to Marah, they could not drink its water because it was bitter. . . . So the people grumbled against Moses, saying, "What are we to drink?" Then Moses cried out to the Lord, and the Lord showed him a piece of wood. He threw it into the water, and the water became fit to drink. There the Lord issued a ruling and instruction for them, and put them to the test. He said, "If you listen carefully to the voice of the Lord your God and do what is right in his eyes, if you pay attention to his commands and keep all his decrees, I will not bring on you any of the diseases I brought on the Egyptians, for I am the Lord, who heals you." Then they came to . . . twelve springs and seventy palm trees, and they camped there near the water.

—Exodus 15:23–27

THE children of Israel had been delivered from the hand of the pharaoh and generations of slavery in Egypt, yet they questioned God's plan for them and how He would provide for their basic needs. We might question their lack of faith, but at the same time we can identify with them in certain circumstances. Especially when we question God and His provisions where our life and health are concerned.

During their journey, the children of Israel became thirsty. Then they began to complain. When their physical condition overpowered their spirit, they forgot that God had always provided for them. They asked, "Where is God now and why has He brought us to this place to die?" They knew all the attributes of God, yet they questioned Him and began to complain. Their trust was dependent upon their circumstances.

When we complain about our circumstances, the attitudes of our minds and the power of our words fight against the deliverance God has for us. Deliverance from our daily struggles. Deliverance from our sickness and pain. When we complain, we forget that God only has good plans for our lives according to Jeremiah 29:11: "'For I know the plans I have for you,' declares the LORD, 'plans to prosper you and not to harm you, plans to give you hope and a future.'"

Our provision has already been made. We may not see it or even understand it, but it has been made. If your find yourself questioning or complaining, call upon the name of the Lord to sweeten the waters of your soul. He will do so, just as He has promised. Many times we may find ourselves much more eager to complain than to call out to God and believe that He has our provision waiting. Trust Him with the kind of trust that can only come from knowing Him. Listen diligently and obey His voice. Look only to Him for provision for every need.

When we trust Him, we can leave the bitterness behind just as the children of Israel left Marah behind and moved on to a better place, a place of strength. They made their dwelling place beside 12 springs and 70 palm trees, a beautiful oasis that was also part of God's provision.

Many times, especially when it seems I am sick all the time, I find myself camped in the wilderness of discontent, complaining as I begin to pitch my own little tent of self-pity. Yet it does me no good and it can spring up a root of bitterness (Hebrews 12:15) quite quickly. No matter what has come into my life, whether as a result of chronic illness or just life's circumstances, I never want to be bitter. Instead I want to become better. To do that, I have to make a conscious choice to abandon the bitterness and move on to the springs of sweet water the Lord has so graciously provided.

DEAR LORD,

I rebuke bitterness in the name of Jesus. I know the plans You have for me are good and not evil. I make a choice today to become better from this journey, not bitter. But, Lord, I do get weary and fearful. Please help me to praise You whenever I begin to question or complain. Amen.

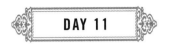

DAY 11

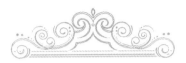

HUGS
FROM GOD

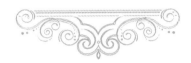

Now let your unfailing love comfort me,
just as you promised me, your servant.

—Psalm 119:76 NLT

I LOVE hugs. I hug everybody! I have even been known to go up to young soldiers and ask them if I can hug them and pray for them. That may seem crazy, but my son is in the Army and when he is far away I cannot hug him myself. I pray for moms all over the world to pray for and love on my son in my absence. Unfortunately, due to all the antibiotics I am on so much of the time, I have a lowered immune system. During cold and flu season, I have to be careful about hugging people because they may have been exposed to something that they pass on to me unknowingly. I have had to stay away from church during the worst of flu season because where I live, in the South, hugging is an automatic instinct.

Many years ago when my boys were young, I was in the hospital. One day I got on the elevator with the most beautiful little boy who had the biggest grin I had ever seen. As the door closed and I spoke to him and his mom, I noticed that he had been burned quite extensively all over his little body. Even though he experienced great pain, his smile was infectious and his giggle contagious. He anxiously awaited his floor so he could return to his room and eat the cheese curls and candy he held in his little burned hands. As he and his mom exited the elevator, tears rolled down my cheeks. How I missed my boys! At that moment I knew I had just been hugged by God. The joy I felt from that precious boy warmed my heart and gave me encouragement until I was home again. There have been many times in my life when I have felt those same hugs from God.

Not long ago I was really missing my daddy, whom I lost in 2007. I had not expressed this to anyone, not even my husband. Our grandson was visiting, and he and my husband were teasing each other about feet. Then, in a very serious, sweet voice, my grandson told "Big-Daddy" that he would rub his feet if he wanted. He walked over, removed his grandfather's socks and began to rub his feet as they continued to tease each other. Only God knew that I used to take my daddy's socks off and rub his feet for a "yankee dime" (a kiss). I had to leave the room before they noticed the tears flowing from my heart onto my face. I whispered a "Thank You, God" as I dried my tears.

Oh, how I love hugs. Especially hugs from God! Living with chronic sickness, pain, or depression can cause us to long for hugs from God. Often when I am feeling down, someone will come along and hug me and I know it was a hug sent from above. That always make me smile, and most of the time I will shed a tear of thanks. God's hugs remind us of His comfort and unfailing love for us.

Do you need a hug from God today? Chances are you are getting them all the time, but you do not recognize what they are. Maybe you live alone or are alone in the hospital right now, and you just need that feeling of a touch from God. I pray that right now, wherever you are, in whatever state of mind or with whatever physical need you have, you will receive a hug from God.

DEAR LORD,

Thank You for Your hugs today. Help me to recognize Your hugs and give You praise for every one. Just as we love our children, Lord, and we long to feel them in our arms, so do You long to hold me as Your child. Thank You for Your hugs, today and every day. Amen.

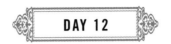

DAY 12

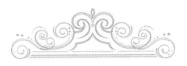

THE STIGMA
OF DEPRESSION

*A happy heart makes the face cheerful,
but heartache crushes the spirit.*

—Proverbs 15:13

I AM seeing the need, as I age, to adapt to my changing health status. My so-called normal is not achievable anymore. I tire much easier and lose optimum health faster. It also takes a little longer to recover when I get sick, and even then the health status I reach is not up to what I would like. Due to my declining health, I am now faced with the necessity of a double lung transplant. Having said all that, I am so thankful for the health I have and the quality of life that I live. Praise God for His mercy and grace! However, I do still get down sometimes. I make it a constant prayer not to allow depression to become my constant state of mind.

Several years ago I attended a women's conference where one of the highlighted speakers was a well-known singer and author. She talked about depression—not just having the blues now and then, but real clinical depression. When she spoke, I felt as though she was talking to me. I had begun taking medication for depression the year that my dad died. But I constantly was trying to get off the medication due to the stigma attached to taking anti-depressants. That weekend, the Lord used that woman to speak into my spirit, and I felt released from the self-imposed need to stop taking the medication. She spoke about how women go to the doctor for physical needs, but when we are in the midst of the darkness that is depression, we try to ignore it. We just smile more, suck it all in, and tell ourselves we are—or should be—happy. What she spoke about brought freedom for me. Depression is no different than physical illness. Sometimes we need medication.

I had been walking around with this cloud over my head, allowing the enemy to stifle me and even bring on a darker place of depression. I kept telling myself that I was OK, I had no reason to be sad or down, and I just needed to pull myself together, put on a smile, and stop crying so much.

Despite my history of illness—understand, chronic illness—I viewed depression in a different light. I felt ashamed. I didn't want anyone to know how I felt, much less that I had been prescribed medication to help with it. I never thought of physical illness having a certain stigma to it but, in my mind, depression did. Through God's amazing grace and compassion, He spoke to me that weekend in the midst of thousands of women. I felt as though He had whispered to my spirit, "Listen up, this is for you, now you are free from the bonds that you have allowed to be placed on you."

To this day I walk in that freedom, just as thankful for the medications that help level out my emotions as I am for the ones that help my CF. Praise God for His supply for *all* our needs!

If you suffer from depression, don't allow it to be a noose around your neck. Instead, allow God to walk you through this time in your life for His glory. He promises not to leave us nor forsake us (Hebrews 13:5).

No matter the situation, whether He chooses to deliver you from that darkness supernaturally or with medication, do not place a stigma on yourself and certainly do not allow anyone else to put that stigma on you, either. God is in control and, no matter your life circumstances and the consequences thereof, "This too shall pass!"

DEAR LORD,

I give You my entire being, mind, soul, and body. I bind the stigma of depression; I want to be free to be all You created me to be. Thank You, Lord, for supplying all my needs according to Your riches in glory through Christ Jesus. May my life, in all circumstances, bring glory and honor to You. Amen.

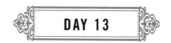

DAY 13

DOWN BUT NOT DISCOURAGED

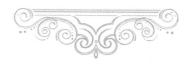

When anxiety was great within me,
your consolation brought me joy.

—Psalm 94:19

WHEN I am hospitalized for an extended stay, 14–30 days, it is usually because my doctor is attempting to control the infection in my lungs by using high-powered antibiotics. They also increase the chest physical therapy that I do at home every day. The multiple aerosols and chest therapy are to loosen the thick mucus that my body overproduces, in order for me to be able to cough it up and out! These hospital stays are difficult because I am not the kind of person who likes to slow down. I also hate having to be away from my family. However, I am reminded each time I am in the hospital that I am blessed to enjoy the level of health I have at my age and lived to be 48 when doctors predicted I would not live to be three. Medical science has certainly progressed over the years, but I give all the praise, honor, and glory to God.

When I have to be in the hospital, my grandchildren come to visit. We play volleyball across the bed with a blown-up surgical glove. I let them ride on my IV pole. We go to the gift shop and they buy candy. We make the best of the situation. My oldest grandson, now 12, has been coming to visit me from the time he was six months old. He feels almost as at home in a hospital room as he does at my real home. It may not be the way I would have wanted it, but this is my life and what a beautifully sweet life it is.

Recently I joined an online panel of adult CF patients who share our CF stories and how it affects our daily lives. We do this in order to encourage others. After posting my story, I stated, "Cystic fibrosis does not define my life, rather it is merely a small part of an amazing journey that I am on."

Of course, some days still hold surprises. Actually, many days hold surprises when you live with chronic illness. Even in the midst of those surprises, I remind myself that this is my journey and that God's plan is perfect as well as His timing. Along this journey I love to see how God chooses to show Himself to me in and through this disease. I am learning to embrace each day, with all its challenges, and just look forward to what is next. His love, mercy, and grace never cease to amaze me.

Your circumstances, physically or otherwise, may cause you to be down at times or even down often. However, don't be discouraged. Maybe your journey is different and seemingly more difficult than someone else's. That gives you more opportunities to encourage yourself in the Lord. Make yourself available to be used by Him as you encounter others along your journey.

DEAR LORD,

I pray You will speak to my spirit when I feel down. Remind me that I have been blessed beyond measure with Your love, Your mercy, Your grace, and Your Holy Spirit. Lord, I pray that not only will I be encouraged but that I will also be used to encourage others. I may get down at times, but I will not let that discourage me or defeat me. Amen.

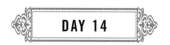

DAY 14

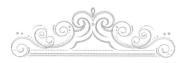

IT'S NOT ABOUT ME

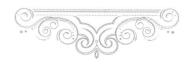

My old self has been crucified with Christ.
It is no longer I who live, but Christ lives in me.
So I live in this earthly body
by trusting in the Son of God,
who loved me and gave himself for me.

—GALATIANS 2:20 NLT

I T's all about me," was the opening line of a popular song. That is how most of the world views life and how they think everyone else should view life. What we seem to have difficulty understanding is that it is *not* about us at all. No matter our physical state or our mental state. Our focus should not and cannot be on ourselves.

Several years ago I went to summer camp with our church youth. The camp theme was, "It's all about *me*." The entire week was focused on how the world teaches us to focus on ourselves because, after all, no one else will. But, the world's philosophy is wrong. That week the youth learned it was all about God and not themselves. The *me* was really *He!* The camp caused them to question what life is really about. *Do* we have a purpose? Why? What is my purpose?

When living with chronic illness, pain, depression, or any other ongoing medical condition, there is a lot of attention placed on you as the patient. It would be very easy to develop the attitude of "it's all about me" and to question: Why me? Why now? Why this? Even amid hurt and struggles, our mind must be on the Lord.

The one and only person who ever walked the face of the earth and possibly could have claimed that it was all about Him was Jesus Christ, yet He did not. Jesus spent His entire earthly ministry proclaiming that it was not at all about Him but all about God, His father, the one that sent Him. How eager He was to please His father and to accomplish the mission that He was sent to earth to do. Even as Jesus hung on the Cross, He knew it was not about Him and He prayed to His father in heaven to forgive those whose hands had been covered in His blood (Luke 23:34).

"It's all about Me," says the God that created us in His image and lovingly provided all we will ever need in this life. He is not surprised by your health or lack of health. He has showered us with His love, mercy, and grace and they are each far beyond our comprehension. "It's all about Me" means that God loved us so much that before the foundation of the world was laid, He had a plan and a purpose for my life and for your life. He even gave the life of His own Son to accomplish that plan in each of our lives. It's all about Him because He designed us with the desire to have a relationship with Him. It's all about Him because He desires and deserves our love and worship.

In the midst of your daily struggles, remember it's not at all about you and your circumstances. It is all about God and how you embrace Him despite the circumstances in your life. When we yield our entire being to Him and allow Him to use us where we are, our focus will change from inward to upward.

DEAR LORD,

Please forgive me when I think more of myself than of You. I pray that today I would keep my mind on the things above and not concentrate on my health or circumstances. Just as You gave Your life for me, Lord, I give my life to You and desire to live in a way to honor You and point others to You. Amen.

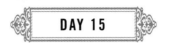

DAY 15

JUST GO
WITH IT

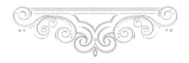

We can make our plans,
*but the L*ORD *determines our steps.*

—P<small>ROVERBS</small> 16:9 NLT

L IVING with chronic illness and all the unplanned fallout that comes with that, there are many things I cannot control or change, so I change what I can—my hair. My husband laughs at me and jokes about my changing hair. I am constantly cutting and coloring it differently. I rarely have the same style for more than three to six months. With all that CF has done to my body, I always joke about my hair being the *one* thing I can control!

I look forward to summer, not for the heat, but because our grandchildren get to spend a lot of time with us. I always try to plan ahead a little and have a short hospital stay (I call it a "tune-up") to prepare for all the activities ahead. Due to my health status declining in the past few years, my plans have not always worked out as I would have liked. Recently we had plans for an entire summer full of activities, trips, and swimming. I was so excited. While the temperatures were still mild, suddenly the humidity became intense, causing my breathing to be difficult. My fun, summer outdoor activities went out the window. Next I got so sick I was unable even to go outside. Then my asthma kicked into high gear, and just getting around *inside* the house became a struggle. *Bummer!*

I thought back to the year before, when I had been able to stay outside, swimming and playing all summer. Our entire family went to the beach for a week. We made sweet memories for all of us, five generations. Of course, we had planned all of it, but in reality we had little control over how it would happen or even if it would happen.

Unlike the summer that all went as planned, many of the activities I normally enjoy have been delayed—or even cancelled—lately. Circumstances beyond our control will cause us to change our plans at times. Often we are disappointed by having to change or cancel things, especially when it's due to our health; however, part of our distress is due to the fact that we do not see the big picture. We are not aware of what God is doing on our behalf behind the scenes.

Maybe your summers, vacations, or just daily routine of life will not be filled with the plans and activities you hope for, but God is so good to give us just what we *need*, even when we plan for something different. It is not wrong for us to make plans, but it is wrong to leave God out of our plans. James put it this way:

Look here, you who say, "Today or tomorrow we are going to a certain town and will stay there a year. We will do business there and make a profit." How do you know what your life will be like tomorrow? Your life is like the morning fog—it's here a little while, then it's gone. What you ought to say is, "If the Lord wants us to, we will live and do this or that." —James 4:13–15 NLT

Take life as it comes and be thankful in everything. You may be pleasantly surprised sometimes, disappointed at others, but God will bless you and bring you joy when you least expect it. Make plans, but give Him your plans. Then be ready to go with His plans. After all, it is the Lord who directs your steps.

DEAR LORD,

You know my heart and my mind better than I do myself. I pray that as I plan my day today and every day You will be my guide. I give my plans to You and yield myself to all You have for my life. I ask forgiveness for when I get angry or question why my plan does not go as I wanted. I thank You for this day and I surrender it to You. Amen.

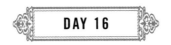

DAY 16

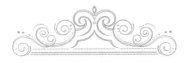

JOY FOR
THE JOURNEY

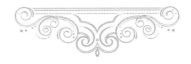

Restore to me the joy of your salvation
and grant me a willing spirit, to sustain me.

—PSALM 51:12

I've got *joy, joy, joy, joy down in my heart. Down in my heart to stay.* I love this song and I love the word *joy.* I can name many things that bring me joy: my marriage, my family, my grandchildren, my friendships. Sometimes joy comes in big outward demonstrations and other times it is in the quiet moments shared between two hearts. Memories can open the floodgates of joy. I believe you can laugh without really knowing the gift of joy but you cannot experience real joy in your life without the outward expression of laughter. Oh, how joy bubbles up from within, again and again!

I love to laugh! When I laugh in public, it always brings on stares because it tends to make me cough. When I cough, people turn around. I cough so hard that I turn beet red and the veins in my neck and face stick out. Women with children are hurrying them away as fast as they can, like I am some walking horror show. Or maybe they think I have a contagious disease. I especially get looks when I am in line somewhere in a crowd. If I get tickled at something, I begin to cough and the person in front of me gives one of those half turns with their eyes cut as far in my direction as they can while trying not to appear like they are looking at me. I know they really want to move as far away from me as possible and bathe in disinfectant.

Thinking of how my coughing unnerves people makes me want to tell them—when I can recover my breath— "Hey . . . this is nothing. A real coughing spell will bring on snorts, sniffs, and spits!" Now that will clear a restaurant quickly. It used to bother me, but I've learned to find humor in it. I just try not to embarrass my grandchildren. They are usually the cause for the laughing hyena fits that lead to embarrassing coughing, choking, and gasping for air. What joy!

Thirteen years ago when I got married, the big joke was that my husband was not getting all of me. I have had many surgeries and most of them were to remove something. I have had part of my intestines removed and my gallbladder, as well as a hysterectomy, a radical mastectomy, an appendectomy, etc. So when we talked about our vows, I promised to give my husband all of me . . . or at least what was still left of me. Since our marriage I have had other surgeries, I am looking at a double lung transplant, and I am sporting a new button peg feeding tube, which means I have detachable parts. I told him if those new lungs are perfect, I will feel like the bionic woman. Breathing easy! Oh, the joy, joy, joy!

I know that many times it is difficult to feel joy when you are struggling from day to day. Joy is a gift of grace! We can spread joy to others just as we can laughter. I love to laugh. I love to make others laugh, but even more importantly, I love to bring joy into others' lives. Joy is beautiful.

Being able to find joy in everything in life can lift not only your spirits but the spirits of those around you. Many times when things are the most difficult, God presents an opportunity to draw from that well of joy that is deep within my heart. Joy is the salve that soothes our hurt and brokenness. I am so thankful for the gift of joy for this journey we call life.

DEAR LORD,

Thank You for Your joy unspeakable at times, which bubbles up from deep inside and causes me to laugh. Thank You for Your gifts of joy and laughter. May I always draw from the joy within when situations and circumstances attempt to steal it. May Your joy be ever present in my life, and may I be faithful to share it with others. Amen.

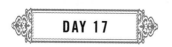

DAY 17

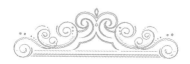

A CHEERFUL
HEART

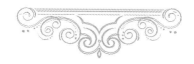

A cheerful heart is good medicine,
but a broken spirit saps a person's strength.

—Proverbs 17:22 NLT

ANY times when things have been the most difficult, God has blessed me with the ability to laugh at my circumstances. Thankfully, He also blessed me with parents and a husband who have the ability to laugh in the midst of the storms.

I never do anything halfway. If I am going to have a problem or an issue it will usually be worst-case scenario. For years I dubbed myself the "Murphy's law" patient. What could go wrong usually did go wrong with me. I figure you can look at that one of two ways, either always be anxious and upset, or adapt the attitude that God just likes to use me to show up and show out. Because no matter what goes wrong—or how wrong it goes—God always gets the victory!

Because the frequency and length of my hospital stays has been increasing, my husband and I seem to go a little stir crazy after about two weeks. We find more to laugh about than you could imagine possible, and we find ways to have fun with the staff. We dress up and do goofy stuff to pass the time. Recently, I was very sick. As I started feeling better, David came up with an idea that we could use camera tricks to make me look like I was shrinking. We took pictures all over the hospital, with nurses, doctors, and each other. We had so much fun doing it, but the response we got from the staff, family, friends, and on Facebook was the best part. We realized that our attitude was contagious and was soon reflected in those caring for me. Now every time I am in the hospital the staff asks, "What are you two going to do to entertain us this time?"

I had to be hospitalized recently for an intestinal blockage. This began out of state so we joke about me having to have the royal treatment and be escorted from Gatlinburg, Tennessee, to Birmingham, Alabama. I spent the first half of that stay trying to break loose the "log-jam" and the second half of the stay trying to stop the dam. I told the nurses that I went from needing dynamite to diapers. Finally I just desperately wanted a cork! They laughed and commented on my positive attitude and outlook. My response is always the same: might as well laugh at it all, it sure beats crying!

We all have struggles. Your struggles may be much harder than another person's. But no matter what you face daily, try to look on the bright side. Look for the humor in the hurt; there usually is some. A cheerful heart really does do good like a medicine!

DEAR LORD,

Although today may not bring much to laugh about, please help me to see the humor in life. I look to You for my cheerful heart. I pray to bring glory to You as Your joy contagiously affects others. May they recognize You and Your joy in me. Amen.

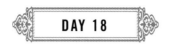

DAY 18

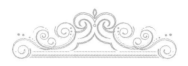

LIVE LIFE TO THE FULLEST

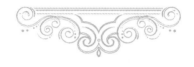

*The thief's purpose is to steal and kill and destroy.
My purpose is to give them a rich and satisfying life.*

—JOHN 10:10 NLT

B ALANCE has never been easy for me. I tend to go all out until I hit a wall, recoup, and then go full force again. This has been a point of contention between my husband and me. Unlike me, he is much better at pacing himself, saying no to people, and not overloading his plate. (As in most marriages, opposites attracted.)

One of the benefits of living with CF is that I have never taken life for granted. I believe this is a true blessing. My motto has always been, "Live life to the fullest!" I believe in cramming everything you can into every minute of every day. I don't put any restrictions on my body, but in the last two years, I've found my body putting more and more restrictions on me. And I don't like that at all! Yet, even when in the hospital, I can live a full and happy life.

Even though we have to change or cancel travel plans due to sickness or me being in the hospital, we make those plans anyway. I definitely believe in having things to look forward to, goals, and aspirations. It makes me push a little harder to stay well or get well enough to enjoy what we have planned. In the same way, we have spent as much time as possible with our grandchildren. I never take for granted the time I have with them. I try to do something every day to make memories for them and for me. Life is but a vapor (James 4:14), even when you are healthy; but when living with chronic illness, it seems to be forever in the forefront. How blessed I am to live the life that I do!

Those living with sickness or pain seem to fall into two categories: they feel they have no real life left or they (like me) feel they cannot take a moment for granted, and they live every one to the absolute fullest. Making memories. Laughing. Loving.

Whatever your challenges are, whether sickness, pain, or depression, God wants you to live your life to the fullest. You may need to be creative at times, but make the effort. Make memories for yourself and your family. Memories are amazing and can carry you, as well as your family, through some of the toughest times in life. Pray that as you live your life fully, you make a profound impact on all those you encounter. May your attitude and passion for life challenge them as well.

However long our moments are here on earth, we are to *enjoy* each one to the *fullest*. Embrace each moment *in joy!*

DEAR LORD,

May I live my life according to the plan You have for me. Lord, I pray that each day I would be mindful of changes I need to make in my life. May I no longer settle for living mundanely due to my circumstances. Your joy is my strength; may it be increased daily as well as the joy in my family. As I wish to honor You with my life, I also desire to inspire others. I give You thanks and praise for my life, for every day and every blessing! Amen.

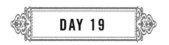

DAY 19

STRENGTH
FOR TODAY

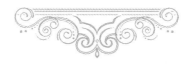

The LORD is my strength and my song;
he has given me victory.

—PSALM 118:14 NLT

THERE have been many times when I have been sick over the years when I have needed real help because I was incapable of helping myself. With even the most basic needs. It never fails, though, that even though I am in great need of help, I think I can handle things myself. I cannot tell you how many times I have gotten out of bed to go to the bathroom and just as I think I can do it, I feel the room spin. Then I hear, "Beth . . . what are you doing? You can't do that by yourself!" I feel help swoop in on both sides of me and rescue me from falling flat on my face. I have always had that "I can do it myself" attitude. And it tends to come out most when I need help the greatest.

I like to watch boxing. I really like it when the guys come into the ring and they look so vastly different. One is usually bigger and more muscular. His opponent may look a little puny, even though they are in the same weight class. Sometimes just a few pounds can make a big difference in their appearance. Some assume that by the looks of the two opponents, the larger is going to win. Then, out of nowhere, the little guy knocks the bigger guy out. I just love it when that happens! It reminds me that it's not the appearance of strength but the actual strength that matters.

By appearance, I am often considered fragile. However, my spirit and my body are strengthened by the Lord. That is where my dependence is. Some days that dependence on His strength is all that gets me through the day, maybe even through each hour of the day.

We often think that we have more strength than we do. We like to think we can handle everything ourselves. We like to feel strong and courageous even when we are not. In times of sickness, hurt, and emotional upsets, we do not have to rely on our own strength or abilities. We have God, who swoops in and raises us up on wings of eagles (Isaiah 40:31). He becomes our victory for us! His strength is our strength and our victory over defeat. In Him we slay sickness, disease, depression, and mental anguish.

Whatever your needs are today, tomorrow, and every day following, God's strength is there for every moment of every day. He lovingly says to you, in essence, "You cannot do this alone. You do not have to do this alone. I am here with you, always, as your strength and your victory!" Even the most basic of needs we think we can handle, we cannot. We must not even attempt. Depend on Him and His strength for today!

DEAR LORD,

Thank You for Your strength. I need You and Your strength today. May I relinquish my do-it-myself attitude and run to Your tower of strength. Thank You that in and through Your strength I have the victory today! Amen.

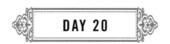

DAY 20

PRAISE IN THE MIDST OF THE STORM

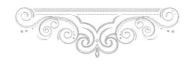

Then God said,
"I am giving you a sign of my covenant
with you and with all living creatures,
for all generations to come.
I have placed my rainbow in the clouds.
It is the sign of my covenant with you
and with all the earth."

—Genesis 9:12–13 NLT

I N THE last year, I have felt like we have been in a storm where my health is concerned. At the beginning of 2014, I was really doing well, and then I began a downward slide when I got pneumonia in the spring. I had to be on oxygen for the first time, except for brief times after surgery or asthma attacks. It was such a struggle to breath at times I thought I would inhale the entire oxygen tube just trying to breathe comfortably. Finally, I was able to be free of the oxygen before going home. Doctors assured me that this was just a momentary lapse and I would be back to normal soon. Little did we know that "normal" for me would be quite different than it had been up to this point in my health.

In the next months, I was hospitalized numerous times, and each time I was unable to reach my previous state of health. I had lost so much weight due to infection that my doctors had a feeding tube placed in my stomach. About this time, I was introduced to the need for a double lung transplant and eventually was sent to Duke in North Carolina to begin the process. Wow, it was quite a year! During it I actually spent more days in the hospital than at home. However, I was out for my grandchildren's birthdays, my wedding anniversary, and a short trip to Gatlinburg, Tennessee, with two of our grands. Plus a wonderful week at the beach in the fall with our closest friends from the United Kingdom. I also managed to be home for Thanksgiving with the family, but then was hospitalized for 31 days, making it home just in time for Christmas.

I praised God every time I was able to enjoy milestones in our lives. No matter how dark things were at times, they always made way for the rainbow. Have you ever noticed that a rainbow seems the most vibrant after the worst of storms? So it is with life. After every storm the rainbow is so brilliant and colorful. A darkened sky just increases the visibility and our appreciation of its beauty.

I know my storms are not over, but I also know that my God is faithful. With every storm, there will be a rainbow. What an awesome God we serve! Just when we think we have had all we can stand, the clouds break and the sun shines through. It's as if God is sending us a hug, to encourage, strengthen, and bless us on our journey.

Not everyone's journey is the same. We know that we will encounter difficulties, storms in life. Sometimes we just have to remind ourselves that God is in control, and He will send that rainbow just when we need it. His timing is perfect. His love is unfailing. Praise Him daily for every blessing and every gift of grace, no matter how small or silly it may seem at the time. Find praiseworthy moments in each day.

Praise Him during the storm and look up. The rainbow is over the horizon. Just wait expectantly!

DEAR LORD,

I pray that no matter what my day may bring, I will praise You. I thank You for the promise of the rainbow because it reminds me of Your faithfulness. May you find me faithful as I honor You each day with my life. I give You praise, honor, and glory in the midst of my storms. Amen.

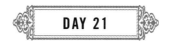

DAY 21

OUR VERY PRESENT HELP

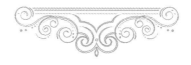

My help comes from the LORD,
who made heaven and earth!

—PSALM 121:2 NLT

R ECENTLY I was admitted to the hospital to undergo treatment for pneumonia. During most hospitalizations, I am mobile and active unless I am undergoing infusions of IV antibiotics. This trip was anything but routine. Soon after admission, my body decided to revolt. My lungs shut down, and I was placed on oxygen. Walking just a few steps exhausted me. I coughed but without any relief for the constant congestion in my chest. I was shocked because I was not that sick when I came in.

After a procedure to take some samples of the mucus directly from my lungs, things went downhill fast. I could see that others were concerned for me when they looked into my eyes. During those days God placed laborers in our pathway to encourage us. We were able to laugh and share the love of family. At every turn, we were met with grace and blessings. Oh what an awesome God we serve! What a doting Daddy to see to our every need, before we were aware of them.

One day when my breathing was really bad and I had that panicky feeling of not being able to get any air into my lungs, I began to think of Psalm 42:1, "As the deer pants for streams of water, so my soul pants for you, my God." I was literally panting for breath in my natural body as my spirit was crying out to God for help. That is the moment I felt His Spirit envelop me. Every time I became short of breath and my oxygen level would drop, I would meditate on that Scripture and realize that, just as He satisfies the deer with water, He would give me oxygen.

My struggles were not only in the physical realm, but also in the spiritual. I knew that I was desperate for God to touch my body, but even more so, I needed Him to soothe my spirit. To give me peace that passes all understanding (Philippians 4:7), to give me His power in my weakness (2 Corinthians 12:9) and, above all else, to glorify Himself. I needed Him to sustain and strengthen my husband, David, and my mom as they cared for me. I did not want them to sense my anxiety. My earnest prayers were uttered in seclusion. My falling tears drenched my spirit. Yet, in my despair He held me close and calmed my fears. I was assured of His tangible presence and His love for me. His grace gathered me to Him as we journeyed down this new, treacherous pathway.

Just as I would begin to faint, Abba, Father, Daddy God would pick me up and carry me, imparting His strength, and the journey continued. I wanted so desperately to be strong, but inside I was scared. It's natural to be scared and confused when facing a health crisis, but we must not take up residence in that state of mind.

When Jesus' disciples failed to stay awake to pray for Him while He was in agony in the Garden of Gethsemane, He told them, "the spirit is willing, but the flesh is weak" (Matthew 26:41). My spirit was willing and knew where to gain strength, but my body was weak. The mind is the battleground that decides whether there will be a victory or defeat in this battle.

I soon found myself on the road to recovery. However, in one way my desperation had not lessened, possibly because I had experienced needing Him more than I ever had. My physical, mental, and emotional struggles continue, but I know where my help comes from. I must stay in the place of total dependence. He will sustain. He always comforts. He longs to be my help.

Whatever your struggles, great or small, whether physical, emotional, or spiritual, remember where your help comes from—run to Him! He is your ever-present help in times of trouble (Psalm 46:1).

DEAR LORD,

Thank You for being my help. May I look only to You, not only when I struggle but in everything. Lord, when others fail me, remind my spirit that You will never leave me nor forsake me. I love You, Lord. Today and every day I need a touch from You, physically, emotionally, and spiritually. Thank You for Your presence and Your love for me. Amen.

30 DAYS OF HOPE

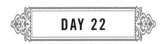

DAY 22

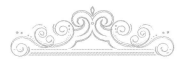

WILL YOU
TRUST ME?

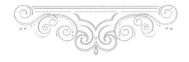

Trust in the LORD with all your heart
and lean not on your own understanding;
in all your ways submit to him
and he will make your paths straight.

—PROVERBS 3:5–6

P SALM 3:5-6 has been my life's verse for as long as I can remember. Even when my relationship with the Lord was not in the place that it should have been, I always remembered this passage. It's strange how something can become so familiar to you that it loses its power. Remember the old adage that "familiarity breeds contempt"?

I could quote my life verse. Whenever I heard it used in a sermon, it would cause me to take special note of the point being made. But in actuality the power had gone out of the meaning for me.

One day I was at my church and strolled into a secretary's office. My attention was drawn to the most amazing picture that I had ever seen. It seemed as though the artist had known my name when he had created it.

The picture was of a young girl with long blonde hair sitting on a swing. The most ominous yet loving hand was holding the rope of the swing. The caption at the top of the picture said, "Will you trust me?" Across the bottom of the picture were the words from Proverbs 3:5–6. At that moment the words that I had claimed for so long took up residence inside me with a new vitality and reality. I realized what the Lord had been urging me toward for years. *Would I trust Him?* With my whole life, every detail, leaving my own plans and leaning totally on Him, trusting that He would guide and direct me to the path He had designed for me.

That question seemed so simple. All the time I thought I had been trusting Him, but in that instant I got it and knew what I had been missing for a long time.

Several weeks later that same picture was given to me. I cherish it just as I do the revelation that I received that day of what it is that the Lord wanted from me. My trust. Not a trust merely in word and symbolism, but true trust from within for every aspect of my life, every moment of every hour of every day.

In my situation it was not a particular thing that the Lord was urging me to trust Him for but the fact that I had not really surrendered to Him. I was still trying to hold my own in certain situations when I felt that I could do it myself. I longed to trust as He wanted me to, but in the natural world that had only brought about disappointment. But on that day I heard Him ask me, *Will you trust Me?*

My answer came quickly. I determined in my heart that yes, I would trust Him with all my heart and no longer lean on my understanding. I would leave all things to Him knowing that He has promised to direct my path. And I knew He would. That day I began a new journey of trust with my Lord.

So, what will it be for you? Will you trust Him? When will you start? Today?

DEAR LORD,

I am so thankful that I can trust You. Please forgive me when I do not or have not trusted in You. I pray that I would be mindful always of how You desire my trust as well as how much You deserve my trust. Amen.

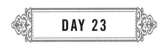

DAY 23

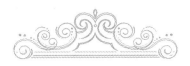

NOT MY WILL

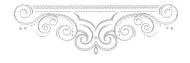

Father, if you are willing,
please take this cup of suffering away from me.
Yet I want your will to be done, not mine.

—LUKE 22:42 NLT

S EVERAL years ago I was in a church service where the guest speaker recounted a family tragedy. They lost their youngest child due to drowning. It was a freak accident. I knew as I sat in that service and listened, God had a poignant lesson for me.

When he was telling about the loss of his child and his family's response, what impacted my spirit so definitely was the statement, "Not my will, but Yours!" Those were the words spoken by his wife. In her darkest moments, the broken, grieving mother, was able to speak this to her heavenly Father, "Not my will, but Yours" . . . "Not my will, but Yours!" How my spirit clung to that phrase. Oh, how my spirit still clings to that phrase. That mother was not questioning God's will; she was completely yielding to God's will. What faith and trust in her God!

Having lost a grandchild at the age of ten months, I, too, have experienced the grief that accompanies the loss of a child. It is a grief very different from that of the loss of an adult, whether friend or family. I remember the cries that were born deep within my spirit. Cries that no words could begin to express! I grieved for our loss as well as for the life that he would not live. Even though I was not the mother, my own pain seemed agonizing, and my questions were endless. Yet, as a mother, I could not begin to imagine or know our daughter's pain. Although the grief was overwhelming, I found comfort in knowing that our precious little one was safe in the arms of Jesus and we would one day be reunited with him. Yet, could I say, "Not my will, but Yours? Not *my* will? But *Yours?*" Lord, "Not my will, but Yours!"

When my daddy, at the age of 65, was dying with cancer, in the midst of my hurt, anger, questions, and fear, could I say, "Not my will, but Yours?" "Not my will? But . . . Yours?" Lord . . . "not my will, but Yours!"

Surrounded by the knowledge and experience of constant sickness, pain, and death in children, teens, and adults living with cystic fibrosis, this disease I know all too well, can I say, "Not my will, but Yours?" "Not my will? But, Yours?" "Lord . . . not my will, but Yours!"

Loss, pain, anger, questions, and disillusionment can all accompany living with chronic illness. Sometimes we find ourselves seeing a side of God we don't understand and really don't like. How does that make us feel? Does it make us question even more? God knows how we hurt, how we question *this* God now being revealed. Yet, how freeing to know that we can come to Him with those feelings, questions, anger, and hurt, and He doesn't reject us.

How do we feel when we are experiencing a side of God that we have not known before? When we are in our darkest times, trials, and tribulations? When we are grieving? When we can't get out of bed due to chronic pain? Do we say, "Not my will? But, Yours?" Or, "Not my will, but Yours!" *Can* we say, "Not my will, but Yours!"?

DEAR LORD,

May we learn of You! May we learn of Your love, Your mercy, and Your grace, so that we can say, no matter the circumstance or situation, "Not my will, but Yours!" May we know You so intimately that we yield to Your will immediately. "Not my will, but Yours!"

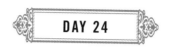

DAY 24

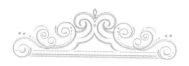

INTERRUPTIONS

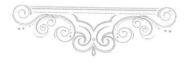

Each time he said, "My grace is all you need.
My power works best in weakness."
So now I am glad to boast about my weaknesses,
so that the power of Christ can work through me.

—2 CORINTHIANS 12:9 NLT

As I mentioned earlier, as my disease progresses, my hospitalizations have become more frequent and longer in duration, often from 21 to 30 days. Now that I am facing a double lung transplant, the stays will become even more frequent and longer.

At one point as an adult, I got very upset about having to be hospitalized so often. I felt like my life was becoming nothing more than sickness and hospitalizations. The Lord spoke to my heart one day and asked me to look at my circumstances differently. My life was amazingly wonderful, filled with love, laughter, and family. He wanted me to recognize that. My life was just interrupted from time to time by complications of CF, sickness, and hospitalizations.

Interruptions. Wow! We get interrupted all the time in everything we do, but I had never thought of my CF as being just an interruption in my life. It made sense. I had certainly not planned my life around this disease. CF was simply part of my life—admittedly a big part—but it did not define me.

I was talking with a mom of a newly diagnosed child with CF. She was asking me questions about having to tell him at some point that he was sick. I quickly responded to her that he is not the illness and shouldn't be defined by it. His *normal* may be filled with doctors' visits, breathing treatments, chest therapy, even hospitalizations, but that would be his normal. I explained to her that CF is a major part of my life, but it is not my life. When I think about who I am and how others see me, CF is involved, but that's not what or who I am. I am Beth Evans, wife, mother, daughter, Nana, writer, author, poet, and speaker who just happens to have cystic fibrosis. It is an interruption to my life at times, but it is not my life.

I know several women who struggle with chronic illness and their lives tend to be interrupted from time to time also; however, that does not define them. They do not let that control their living of their lives.

Whatever your health condition may be, whether you live with diabetes, rheumatoid arthritis,, fibromyalgia, lupus, or any other chronic illness, do not allow it to define you. It will bring complications and struggles into your daily life, but look on them as merely interruptions.

God wants you to be defined by who you are *in Him*, not labeled by sickness or disease. When your interruptions seem to be more than you can bear, carry them to Him and place them at His feet. Remember that no matter your situation or circumstance, His grace is more than enough to see you through your daily struggles—as well as your interruptions.

DEAR LORD,

Help me to focus on You each day. When my health tries to weigh me down, remind me that my struggles may bring interruptions into my life but they do not define my life. May I look to You and rely on Your loving grace to see me through. Amen.

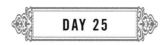

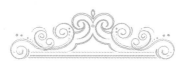

PRAISE, OUR BATTLE CRY

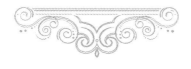

*Early the next morning the army of Judah went out into the
wilderness of Tekoa. On the way Jehoshaphat stopped and said,
"Listen to me, all you people of Judah and Jerusalem!
Believe in the LORD your God, and you will be able
to stand firm. Believe in his prophets, and you will succeed."
After consulting the leaders of the people, the king
appointed singers to walk ahead of the army, singing to the
LORD and praising him for his holy splendor.
This is what they sang: "Give thanks to the LORD;
his faithful love endures forever!"
At the very moment they began to sing and give praise,
the LORD caused the armies of Ammon, Moab, and Mount Seir
to start fighting among themselves.*

—2 CHRONICLES 20:20–22 NLT

I HAVE always cringed when I hear someone refer to me as "suffering from CF." I am not suffering! What I am doing is *battling* CF. I am in a battle for my life, and how I respond to that battle greatly affects the outcome. We have been equipped with weapons of spiritual warfare ensuring our strategic victory in battle. I'm choosing to fight with those weapons.

God told Jehoshaphat to head into battle with praise and songs to the Lord. As they did so, the enemies would set ambushes against each other and would defeat themselves. Praise was to be their battle cry. They were victorious because they led out with praise. The battle belonged to God, not to Judah. The same is true in our lives. The battle belongs to God, not to us. Praise is to be our battle cry. Our strategy. Every day we face a battle. Some days we face many battles. Each day we are to awaken with praise on our lips announcing to the enemy camp that we are ready for battle and that we know the victory is ours.

Psalm 34:1 (NKJV) says, "I will bless the Lord at all times; His praise shall continually be in my mouth." It does *not* say, "when I want to" or "when I feel like it." When my doctor's report is good. When I am having a good day. When I am not depressed. It says "continually" praise will be in my mouth. What a difference it will make today if praise is constantly in our hearts, on our minds, and coming from our mouths. Our praise cannot and must not be conditional.

I know it may be difficult to sing out with praise when your body or your soul is hurting. However, Hebrews 13:15 tells us that with Jesus' help we can constantly offer a sacrifice of praise. Sacrifice! Did you ever think of giving praise to God as a sacrifice?

God knew we would encounter trials and tribulations, struggles. He knew that sometimes it would be a sacrifice for us to praise Him—a sacrifice of time and energy and will. Yet we are encouraged that in and through Christ, we have the help we need and the ability to make that sacrifice. How comforting.

Because breath is so precious to someone with lung disease, I have claimed Psalm 150:6 as another life verse: "Let everything that has breath praise the Lord!" That should be our heart's cry, that praise our battle cry—that we would gain victory in every battle, every day. No battle is too great; nor is any battle too small. Praise must continually be on our lips to the mighty God we serve. He is great and greatly to be praised (Psalm 48:1 NKJV)!

DEAR LORD,

Thank You for my weapons of warfare. Thank You for fighting the battle on my behalf. Thank You for victory over my struggles. Thank You for knowing that my praise would sometimes, even many times, be a sacrifice. Oh God, my God, You are great and greatly will I praise You! Amen.

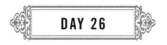

DAY 26

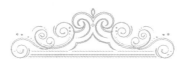

REST IN HIM

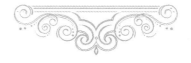

Those who live in the shelter of the Most High
will find rest in the shadow of the Almighty.
*This I declare about the L*ORD*: He alone is my refuge,*
my place of safety; he is my God, and I trust him.

—P*SALM* 91:1–2 NLT

L IVING with chronic illness can bring on many other health-related complications and issues. I call them the fallout of CF or the fallout of fibromyalgia. One of the biggest issues that I have as my lung disease progresses is the inability to sleep well. To fall asleep, I have a bedtime ritual. I take melatonin (an over-the-counter hormone thought to help regulate biorhythms). Then I rub a mixture of essential oils on my feet, pulse points behind my ears, and under my nose. I drink chamomile tea before bed and diffuse a blend of relaxing and sleep-promoting essential oils to help me stay asleep. Even with all that, I may have a hard time going to sleep. If I do go to sleep quickly, I have problems staying asleep. Or I wake in the morning feeling completely unrested.

This lack of restful sleep plays a negative role in my CF and fibromyalgia. With both diseases, I need rest to overcome their complications. Both make it difficult to get that needed rest. This is an ongoing issue that I cannot control.

I remember spending nights with my widowed grandmommy when I was a child. She would lie awake for hours just praying to fall asleep. She told me that she prayed to the Lord to help her fall asleep and that she always added, "I will lay here and rest in You, Lord, until sleep comes." What an awesome way to fall asleep—just resting in Him until sleep comes.

Unlike my grandmommy, if I lie in bed sleepless very long, I get restless and get up and watch TV, write, clean, do laundry, or cook. I have even painted the kitchen while the rest of the household slept. Grandmommy would get a kick out of that! However, I am trying to put into practice Grandmommy's example of rest in and with the Lord until sleep comes. He knows my restlessness, but He deals gently with me and urges me to rest with Him and in Him. Physically as well as spiritually.

When thinking about rest, we often think about getting to bed early, sleeping in, or taking naps. So many times, when illness is such a constant in your life, you need rest for your mind and spirit as much or more than for your body. That is where God is teaching me to slow down and rest in Him. My body needs it, but my spirit also needs it—vitally.

Earlier in this book, I told you about the medications, aerosols, and time-consuming chest physical therapies I take each day. I am also beginning pulmonary rehab at my local hospital that will be an hour each day for three to four days a week but, in the midst of my bodily maintenance, I lead an active, fulfilled life. I have six grandchildren, I am active in my church, and I am an author. Why would anyone think I need rest?

The life I live is truly amazing. Although I may try many remedies to get a restful night's sleep, I find my true rest and solace in Christ and Him alone. All the tea in the world, all the bedtime rituals, the essential oils, and sleep aids are of no effect for my spirit. Only time in the Word, constant conversation with my Lord, and time spent in His peaceful presence will truly allow me to *rest in Him!*

Join me today in practicing the presence of God. Read His Word. Pour your heart out to Him in prayer, and then stay still enough to listen to His response. Learn to rest in Him.

DEAR LORD,

How I need Your rest for my mind, my body, and my spirit. Rest that comes only from Your presence. Lord, teach me to rest in You. When my mind races, remind me to take rest in You. Thank You for Your promise of rest. Amen.

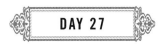

DAY 27

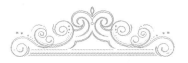

TENACITY

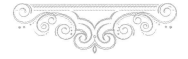

Dear brothers and sisters,
when troubles of any kind come your way,
consider it an opportunity for great joy.
For you know that when your faith is tested,
your endurance has a chance to grow.
So let it grow, for when your endurance is
fully developed, you will be perfect and complete,
needing nothing.

—James 1:2–4 NLT

T ENACITY is a word that has been used to describe my personality and every area of my life, especially when it comes to my attitude toward living with cystic fibrosis. *Tenacious* is an adjective meaning not easily stopped or pulled apart; firm or strong; continuing for a long time; very determined to do something.

My mother will be the first to tell you that from the time of my birth until now "not easily stopped" and "very determined to do something" describe me perfectly. Most people would call me stubborn or bullheaded, but I prefer tenacious. My mother tells stories of how, as a toddler, if I was determined to do something, I did it no matter the consequences. She said she could spank me, and I still would look right in her eyes and do exactly what I had been told not to do. Little did she know at that time how my tenacious spirit would serve me well when it came to living with chronic illness.

Maybe Satan has been trying to take me out from the time of my birth. I was born five weeks premature and weighed only five pounds, one ounce. In 1966 that presented dangers and complications. Only 24 hours after birth, I had surgery to remove 14 inches of my small intestine because it was ruptured. The doctors did not give my parents great hope for my survival. Then at the age of 18 months, I was diagnosed with cystic fibrosis. There have been many bumps, hills, and mountains along the journey since then, but God's grace has seen me through.

Jeremiah was certainly tenacious. In Jeremiah 1, God told Jeremiah that He had put a tenacious spirit in him to face the nation of Judah:

"Today I have made you a fortified city, an iron pillar and a bronze wall to stand against the whole land—against the kings of Judah, its officials, its priests and the people of the land. They will fight against you but will not overcome you, for I am with you and will rescue you," declares the Lord. —Jeremiah 1:18–19

Even though Jeremiah felt inadequate in his abilities, following the leading of God, he stood before Judah with tenacity. However, in Jeremiah 15:10–18, we read that Jeremiah cried out to God in despair, ready to give up. God encouraged him in verses 19–21 by reassuring him that He was with him and would not leave him. Even as a prophet, having been spoken to directly by God, Jeremiah grew weary in his journey, doubted, and just wanted to give up. Wow! Sometimes I forget that all the people in the Bible are just that—people. Ordinary people just like us.

Tenacity is a quality that can serve those of us living with chronic illness well. I like being thought of as having tenacity. Being very determined to do something such as get through the day, fight with everything I have, and not let this disease overcome my spirit.

Do others use the term *tenacious* in describing you? Most people who face struggles every day, whether physical, mental, or emotional, have tenacity. It is a spirit that is evident to those around us. Tenacity and God's grace can be a powerful combination.

DEAR LORD,

Thank You for putting in me the spirit of tenacity. By Your grace, may I be determined today to live to the fullest. When I feel as though I want to give up, please remind me You are with me and will not leave me. May my tenacious spirit glorify You. Amen.

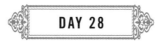

DAY 28

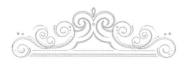

MINISTER
WHERE YOU ARE

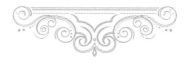

*Jesus came and told his disciples, "I have been given all
authority in heaven and on earth. Therefore, go and
make disciples of all the nations, baptizing them in the
name of the Father and the Son and the Holy Spirit.
Teach these new disciples to obey all the commands
I have given you. And be sure of this:
I am with you always, even to the end of the age."*

—Matthew 28:18–20 NLT

*He said to them, "Go into all the world and
preach the gospel to all creation.
Whoever believes and is baptized will be saved,
but whoever does not believe will be condemned."*

—Mark 16:15–16

W HEN we think of missions, we often think of foreign lands. Or organizations that you support through your local church. We think of missionaries serving in far-away places, in other cultures, speaking other languages. Most of us would agree that when Christ told us to "go into all the world," He literally meant *everywhere.* All the world begins with our surroundings, whatever and wherever that may be. We live on a missions field. We need to be about our Father's business wherever we find ourselves. We need to be salt (Matthew 5:13) and light (1 John 1:7) to a sinful, dark world. We are called to share the love of Christ. There are no limits to when, where, or how we are to share that love.

Although I have to be in the hospital often, I had never thought about it being a missions field for me. However, a very dear, godly man has caused me to look at it differently. When he sends me a note of encouragement or comes for a visit, he reminds me that I am on the missions field. When he prays for me, his prayer always notes the missions field I am called to at present—the hospital. He prays that I have opportunities to share the love and light of Christ while I am there.

My heart's prayer is that I am moldable and usable in every situation. With patients as well as staff, I seek to bring God glory in every aspect of my life. That is what it means to be a missionary: everywhere I go is my missions field.

We all are called to missions. We all live on a missions field. Wherever we live, work, play, and especially where we find others sick and hurting—there are our missions fields. Maybe you take part in a support group. Maybe you can bring encouragement to others in your same situation, physically, mentally, or emotionally. Possibly you have been sent to minister to someone who is giving care to you. You may also be an encouragement to families of others in your situation. You never know where God will use you or how He will use you to minister to others. Where He has placed you, He will use you if you are willing to be used. Just step out in faith! Strike up a conversation, pray with and for someone, send a card, make a visit, or give a reassuring smile or even a hug. Whatever you sense the Lord leading you to do, do it! God's got your back! As you are faithful to bless others, you also will be blessed.

Wherever it may be, go into all *your* world sharing the gospel and the love of Christ!

DEAR LORD,

May I be obedient to minister where You have placed me. As I step out in faith, I know You will guide me. Lord, I desire to spread Your love and Your hope to others in need. May I minister in Your name everywhere I go and to everyone I encounter today. Amen.

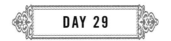

DAY 29

YOU CAN DO IT

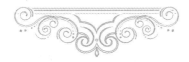

For I can do everything with the help of Christ who gives me strength.

—Philippians 4:13 NLT

M Y OLDEST son is educable mentally retarded, so as he was growing up, we focused on what he *could* do and not the things that were more difficult for him. However, even when we asked things of him that we knew he could do, he would constantly say, "I can't." It broke my heart to hear him say that, but it also made me mad. I knew he could do anything he put his mind to. I knew that the Holy Spirit resided in him and there was nothing beyond His capability.

By the age of seven, he had memorized Philippians 4:13. I claimed that verse for him and taught it to him as his life verse. Whenever he would say, "I can't," I would say, "You what?" Then, on cue, he would recite, "I can do all things through Christ who strengthens me!" To this day if he says, "I can't," I will say, "You what?" and he will recite the verse. (He's 30 now.)

Similarly, as those living with chronic illness, whether mental, physical, or emotional, we can do any and everything in and through Christ's strength. He is how we can push through the days that threaten to pull us under. He is the strength that gets us out of bed, overcomes our anguish, and puts a smile on our face and a song in our heart.

I know personally that there have been more times than I would like to remember that I, too, had to stand on this verse to get myself out of bed, face the day ahead, push through the sickness, depression or pain, and escape the darkness lingering over me disguised as CF or fibromyalgia. It is not easy. But when I think of what may be difficult for me, I remember how my son has struggled all his life. He cannot change his circumstances any more than I can change mine. He brings me such inspiration and such joy. I see how he has pushed through what seemed to be insurmountable odds to graduate high school, get his driver's license, boater's license, and get a job as a painter's apprentice. As an adult he has gone through heart surgery to repair a hole that had probably been there from birth, as well as surgery to remove a benign brain tumor. He is a hero to me! He can do all things, and has done all these things through Christ who gives him strength.

You can do it, too. Be encouraged! You can do all things through Christ who gives *you* strength. Not just some things. Not just the easy things. Not just the things the doctors say you can due to your prognosis. *All things!* You can do all things through Christ who gives you strength! Claim that verse for your life. Never say, "can't" again! "You what?" You can do all things! Yes, you can! You can do *all* things! Through Christ who gives you strength.

DEAR LORD,

I am claiming Philippians 4:13 as my life verse today. I can do all things in and through Your strength. I thank You for the promise of Your strength. I remove the word can't from my vocabulary and my thought processes today. May You alone be glorified in my life and in my strength. Amen.

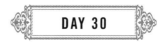

DAY 30

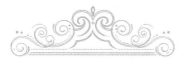

HOPE FOR TOMORROW

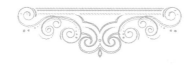

*God did this so that, by two unchangeable things
in which it is impossible for God to lie,
we who have fled to take hold of the hope
set before us may be greatly encouraged.
We have this hope as an anchor for the soul,
firm and secure. It enters the inner sanctuary
behind the curtain, where our forerunner,
Jesus, has entered on our behalf.
He has become a high priest forever,
in the order of Melchizedek.*

—HEBREWS 6:18–20

THIS word *hope* in the Greek means to anticipate, usually with pleasure. Expectation, confidence, and faith. Oh, how encouraging that we have hope for today and forever. Christ Jesus is our hope, our expectation, anticipation, confidence, and faith. What a blessing!

I know that hope is especially needed when living with chronic illness. Even more so if your chronic condition is considered to be terminal, as mine is. I am so thankful that my hope and expectations are not placed on human doctors and man-made medicines. My hope is in Christ. I am so very thankful for my doctors and nurses, as well as the medications, tests and procedures that have improved my quality and length of life. However, that is not where I place my faith and confidence.

As I write this, I am in the process of being listed for a lifesaving double lung transplant at Duke Clinic in Durham, North Carolina. I am so blessed to have the doctor I have in Birmingham who was able to get me sent to Duke. I am also blessed to have the team of doctors who will be making the decisions on my health related to transplant. Yet, my hope is not in them, any of them, nor in the transplant itself. My hope is only in my Lord. He has brought me thus far and I know He will see me through as He brings His plans into place. I will tell you, as thankful as I am to have this option, I feel like Moses when he was having a conversation with God about the future: "The LORD replied, 'My Presence will go with you, and I will give you rest.' Then Moses said to him, 'If your Presence does not go with us, do not send us up from here'" (Exodus 33:14–15).

In other words, Moses was saying, "If You are not going, then I am not going!" Like Moses, who had his hope in God as an anchor for his soul, I do not want to be anywhere other than where God wants me to be, no matter the outcome.

Maybe you are feeling like you have no hope. Maybe you have lost your zest for life due to you illness or circumstances. Remember your hope is in Christ, not man. Whatever the prognosis you may have been given, remember that God is in control of your destiny, not man or disease. Your life and every minute of it has purpose. Look expectantly to every day, consecrating it to God, knowing that in Him—and only in Him—is your hope.

DEAR LORD,

Today I place my hope, all my expectations, in You alone. I refuse to surrender to my illness or circumstances. I want to honor You with my life and the way that others see me live it. I want all that You have for my life and nothing else. I know You alone know my needs and that You alone have already supplied all I ever need. Thank You, Lord, for being my hope, my expectations, and my confidence, not only today but every day of my life. Amen.

Also in the Gifts of Hope series...

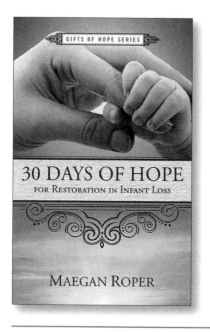

30 Days of Hope for
Restoration in Infant Loss

Maegan Roper

ISBN-13: 978-1-59669-438-5

N154116 · $9.99

30 Days of Hope for Restoration in Infant Loss

by Maegan Roper

Losing an infant through miscarriage, stillbirth, or a birth defect is a heartbreaking and sometimes lonely experience. Author Maegan Roper speaks new hope to the hearts of devastated mothers and fathers in the midst of their loss. With 30 days of Scripture truths that comforted her after her daughter's death, Maegan addresses the chaos parents may feel:

- Is God truly in control?
- How can I ever enjoy life again?
- What is my child's life like in heaven?
- Will the pain ever fade?

In a tender but powerful voice, *30 Days of Hope for Restoration in Infant Loss* insists that God can make things good again—in this life and, especially, in the life to come!

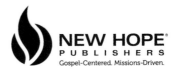

NEW HOPE
P U B L I S H E R S
Gospel-Centered. Missions-Driven.

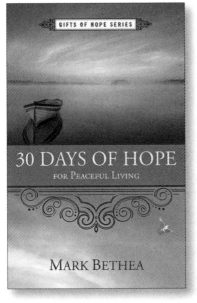

30 Days of Hope for
Peaceful Living

Mark Bethea

ISBN-13: 978-1-59669-437-8

N154115 · $9.99

===

30 Days of Hope for Peaceful Living

by Mark Bethea

Sometimes life seems full of obstacles that can prevent us from experiencing peace in Christ. Even in the safest place life can offer, you can feel devoid of peace. No matter how hard you try, you can't seem to find a peaceful balance of living between your worry over the present and fear of the future.

30 Days of Hope for Peaceful Living offers encouraging insight through examining what God's Word has to say about peace. Author and pastor, Mark Bethea shares biblical understanding for how peaceful living can be accomplished, no matter what life throws at you.

 For information visit **NewHopePublishers.com**